Principles of Pharmacology for Respiratory Care

Student Workbook

GEORGINE W. BILLS, MBA, RRT
ROBERT C. SODERBERG, DDS, MS

Delmar Publishers Inc.™
I(T)P™

NOTICE TO THE READER

Publisher does not warrant or guarantee any of the products described herein or perform any independent analysis in connection with any of the product information contained herein. Publisher does not assume, and expressly disclaims, any obligation to obtain and include information other than that provided to it by the manufacturer.

The reader is expressly warned to consider and adopt all safety precautions that might be indicated by the activities described herein and to avoid all potential hazards. By following the instructions contained herein, the reader willingly assumes all risks in connection with such instructions.

The publisher makes no representations or warranties of any kind, including but not limited to, the warranties of fitness for particular purpose or merchantability, nor are any such representations implied with respect to the material set forth herein, and the publisher takes no responsibility with respect to such material. The publisher shall not be liable for any special, consequential or exemplary damages resulting, in whole or in part, from the readers' use of, or reliance upon, this material.

For information, address

Delmar Publishers Inc.
3 Columbia Circle
Box 15015
Albany, New York 12212-5015

Printed in the United States of America
Published simultaneously in Canada
by Nelson Canada,
a division of The Thomson Corporation

1 2 3 4 5 6 7 8 9 10 XXX 00 99 98 97 96 95 94

ISBN: 0-8273-5275-1
Library of Congress Catalog Card Number: 93-48582

Contents

Answers to the workbook questions can be found in the Instructor's Guide to accompany *The Principles of Pharmacology for Respiratory Care* by Georgine W. Bills and Robert Soderberg.

Part I: General Pharmacologic Principles

CHAPTER 1

General Pharmacologic Concepts

Answer the following questions in your own words. Write your answers in the spaces provided.

1. Why should a respiratory therapist have a general knowledge of all types of drugs and not just respiratory therapy drugs?

____

____

____

____

____

2. Define pharmacology. ______________________________

____

____

What are four categories of pharmacologic study?

a) ______________________________

b) ______________________________

c) ______________________________

d) ______________________________

3. Define the following terms.

a) dose-response curve: ______________________________

____

b) theraputic dose: ______________________________

____

c) lethal dose fifty (LD_{50}) ______________________________

____

d) effective dose fifty (ED_{50}) ______________________________

____

e) theraputic index (TI): ______

______

f) idiosyncrasy: ______

______

g) allergy: ______

______

h) drugs: ______

______

i) placebo: ______

______

j) tolerance: ______

______

k) theraputic effect: ______

______

l) tachyphylaxes: ______

______

m) side effect: ______

______

n) drug nomenclature: ______

______

1) chemical name: ______

2) generic name: ______

3) trade (proprietary) name: ______

o) toxic effect: ______

p) teratogen: ______

q) carcinogen: ______

r) drug dependence: ______

4. Describe the basic structure and chemical makeup of the cell membrane.

______

______

______

Define:

a) bilipid: ______________________________

____

b) integral proteins: ______________________________

____

c) channel: ______________________________

____

d) fluid mosaic model: ______________________________

____

5. Describe the difference between mechanism of action and site of action.

mechanism of action: ______________________________

____

____

____

site of action: ______________________________

____

____

____

6. In general terms, describe a receptor site. ______________________________

____

What is the difference between an agonist and an antagonist?

agonist: ______________________________

____

antagonist: ______________________________

____

7. Briefly describe the five main physiological factors that affect the action of drugs.

a) route of administration: ______________________________

____

b) absorption: ______

______

c) distribution: ______

______

______

e) excretion: ______

______

8. With respect to absorption of drugs, discuss the importance of lipid solubility and drug ionization.

lipid solubility: ______

______

______

drug ionization: ______

______

______

______

9. With respect to drug metabolism, explain what is meant by microsomal enzyme induction.

______

______

______

______

10. Explain how patient compliance, pathological state, and drug interaction might alter the effects of a drug.

patient compliance: ______

______

______

pathological state: ______

______

______

drug interaction: ______

______

______

CHAPTER 2

Pharmacology of the Autonomic Nervous System

Answer the following questions in your own words. Write your answers in the spaces provided.

1. Compare the difference in function between the somatic, sympathetic, and parasympathetic nervous systems.

   somatic nervous system: ______________________________

   ____

   ____

   ____

   sympathetic nervous system: ______________________________

   ____

   ____

   ____

   parasympathetic nervous system: ______________________________

   ____

   ____

   ____

2. Define the term neurotransmitter. ______________________________

   ____

   ____

   ____

   Indicate the neurotransmitter released at the neuroeffector site in the sympathetic and parasympathetic division of the ANS.

   sympathetic division ______________________________

   ____

   parasympathetic division ______________________________

   ____

3. List the overall effects of the sympathetic nervous system on the following.

a) arteries: ____

____

b) heart: ____

____

c) gastrointestinal tract: ________________________________

____

d) pupil of the eye: __________________________________

____

e) respiratory tract: __________________________________

____

f) urinary bladder: __________________________________

____

4. List the names of the receptors in the sympathetic division of the ANS and the general locations where these receptors can be found.

Names:	Locations:
a) ____________________	a) ____________________
b) ____________________	b) ____________________
c) ____________________	c) ____________________

5. Describe the overall effects of α-adrenergic drugs.____________________________

____

____

____

List three examples of these drugs: a) _______________ b) _______________ c) _______________

6. Describe the overall effects of β-adrenergic drugs.____________________________

____

____

____

List three examples of these drugs.

a) ______

b) ______

c) ______

7. Describe the overall effects of α-blocking drugs. ______

______

______

______

Give one example of this type of drug. ______

8. Describe the overall effects of β-blocking drugs. ______

______

______

______

Give three examples of these drugs.

a) ______

b) ______

c) ______

9. Describe the overall effects of the neuronal activators and blocking drugs. ______

______

______

______

What is their main clinical use? ______

______

10. Describe the overall effects of the parasympathetic division of the ANS.

______

______

______

11. List the names of the receptors in the parasympathetic division of the ANS and the general locations where the receptors can be found.

Names:	Locations:
a) ______	a) ______
b) ______	b) ______
c) ______	c) ______

12. Describe the overall effects of the choline esters. ______

______

______

______

Give two examples of these drugs.

a) ______

b) ______

13. Describe the overall effects of the anticholinesterase drugs. ______

______

______

______

Give one example of these drugs. ______

14. Describe the overall effects of the anticholinergic drugs. ______

______

______

______

Give three examples of these drugs.

a) ______

b) ______

c) ______

15. Why is acetylcholine *not* used clinically as a drug?

CHAPTER 3

Pharmacology of the Central Nervous System

Answer the following questions in your own words. Write your answers in the spaces provided.

1. Why are action drugs in the CNS so hard to predict in terms of site of action and mechanism of action?

____

____

____

____

____

2. List and describe six general characteristics of CNS drugs.

a) ______________________________

____

b) ______________________________

____

c) ______________________________

____

d) ______________________________

____

e) ______________________________

____

f) ______________________________

____

3. Define the term sedative. ______________________________

____

____

Define the term hypnotic. ______________________________

____

____

4. What are the overall effects of barbiturates? ______________________________

____

____

____

List the main clinical uses of barbiturates. ______________________________

____

5. Describe the overall mechanism of action of the benzodiazepines. ______________________________

____

____

Why has this group of drugs become the primary drug group used in the treatment of anxiety? ______________

____

____

6. Why is alcohol perceived sometimes as an excitatory drug rather than a depressant drug?

____

____

____

7. Define the term psychopharmacology.

____

____

What is the rationale behind the drugs in the treatment of mental and behavioral disorders?

____

____

8. List the seven categories of psychopharmacologic agents and the type of psychiatric disorders that are treated by each drug.

Categories:

a) ______

b) ______

c) ______

d) ______

e) ______

f) ______

g) ______

Psychiatric disorders:

a) ______

b) ______

c) ______

d) ______

e) ______

f) ______

g) ______

9. Describe the overall effect that the discovery of phenothiazine drugs had on the treatment of psychosis.

______

______

______

______

10. Describe the chemical basis for drugs used to treat various types of depression.

______

______

______

______

11. Describe the mechanism of action of the MAOI and TCA antidepressant drugs.

______

______

______

Why do MAOI drugs need to be monitored carefully? ______

______

______

12. List three examples of the new generation of the antidepressants.

a) ______________________________

b) ______________________________

c) ______________________________

Why are these drugs more popular than the MAOI and TCA antidepressants?

____

____

____

13. List two diseases that are treated by mood stabilizing drugs.

a) ______________________________

____

b) ______________________________

____

14. List two main clinical uses of psychostimulant drugs.

a) ______________________________

b) ______________________________

What is the paradoxical effect of these drugs in treating hyperactivity?

____

____

15. Which drugs are currently the most frequently used antianxiety agents?

a) ______________________________

b) ______________________________

c) ______________________________

d) ______________________________

e) ______________________________

16. What drugs are used to treat the following clinical diseases?

Diseases:	Drugs:
Tourette's syndrome	a) ______
panic attack	b) ______
nocturnal enuresis	c) ______

17. Define the term epilepsy. ______

______

What two drugs are used often to treat generalized grand mal seizures and petit mal seizures?

generalized grand mal:

a) ______

b) ______

petit mal:

a) ______

b) ______

18. What causes parkinsonism? ______

______

______

______

Why is the drug L-dopa the most effective treatment? ______

______

______

______

19. Define the term general anesthesia. ______

______

______

List five properties of an ideal general anesthetic.

a) ______________________________

b) ______________________________

c) ______________________________

d) ______________________________

e) ______________________________

20. Explain why anesthesiologists use a combination of drugs when administering a general anesthetic agent.

____

____

____

____

21. In terms of classifications of general anesthetics, complete the following.

List one example of a gas. ______________________________

List two examples of a volatile liquid.

a) ______________________________

b) ______________________________

List two examples of an IV agent.

a) ______________________________

b) ______________________________

22 Briefly discuss advantages of IV general anesthetics as opposed to the use of a volatile liquid or gas combination.

____

____

____

____

23. Discuss the rationale for the administration of preanesthetic agents prior to the administration of general anesthetics.

____

____

____

24. Define the term narcotic. ______________________________

____

____

____

Discuss the mechanism of action of narcotics. ______________________________

____

____

25. Describe the effects of narcotics on the following systems of the body.

CNS: ______________________________

____

respiratory system: ______________________________

____

GI tract: ______________________________

____

26. Complete the following according to the classification of narcotics. List two examples from the classification of agonist, two examples from agonist/antagonist, and one example from antagonist.

agonist:

a) ______________________________

b) ______________________________

agonist/antagonist:

a) ______________________________

b) ______________________________

antagonist:

____

27. Describe the important clinical use of Naloxone.

____

____

____

____

28. Using salicylates as the prototype nonnarcotic analgesic, list five therapeutic uses.

a) ____________________

b) ____________________

c) ____________________

d) ____________________

e) ____________________

29. Describe one advantage and one disadvantage of the use of acetaminophen.

advantage: ____________________

____

disadvantage: ____________________

____

30. What is the major clinical use of nonsteroidal anti-inflammatories? ____________________

____

What are their main adverse effects? ____________________

____

CHAPTER 4

Skeletal Muscle Relaxants

Answer the following questions in your own words. Write your answers in the spaces provided.

1. Compare the mechanism of action between the tree types of peripheral-acting muscle relaxants and list one example of each type of drug.

Mechanism of Action	Peripheral-Acting Muscle Relaxants
a) ____________________	a) ____________________
b) ____________________	b) ____________________
c) ____________________	c) ____________________

2. Why should nondepolarizing and depolarizing muscle relaxants only be used by an anesthesiologist, or those who are specifically trained in the use of these drugs?

____

____

____

3. What is the main advantage of using the direct-acting peripheral muscle relaxants?

____

____

____

____

4. What is the main therapeutic effect of the CNS muscle relaxants?

____

____

____

____

CHAPTER 5

Cardiovascular and Renal Pharmacology

Answer the following questions in our own words. Write your answers in the spaces provided.

1. Define the term automaticity. ______________________________

____

Correlate the conduction system of the heart to a normal ECG. ______________________________

____

P-wave means: ______________________________

____

QRS means: ______________________________

____

T-wave means: ______________________________

____

2. Briefly describe the overall effects of congestive heart failure with regard to heart enlargement and accumulation of edema fluid.

____

____

____

____

3. Define the following terms.

a) arteriosclerosis: ______________________________

____

b) angina pectoris: ______________________________

____

c) myocardial infarction: ______________________________

____

4. Describe the overall clinical effects of the cardiac glycosides.

____

____

____

____

5. List three clinical effects of digitalis and four adverse effects.

clinical effects:

a) ____

b) ____

c) ____

adverse effects:

a) ____

b) ____

c) ____

d) ____

What is digitalization? ____

____

____

6. Define the term arrhythmia. ____

____

Compare the difference between supraventricular arrhythmias and ventricular fibrillation.

supraventricular: ____

____

____

ventricular fibrillation: ____

____

____

7. List three of the four reasons for converting cardiac arrhythmias.

a) ______________________________

b) ______________________________

c) ______________________________

8. List the four classifications of antiarrhythmic drugs and give at least one example of each classification.

Classifications	Examples of Drugs
a) ______________	a) ______________
b) ______________	b) ______________
c) ______________	c) ______________
d) ______________	d) ______________

9. Define angina pectoris. ______________________________

____

Describe the overall effects of antianginal drugs in terms of relieving pain. ______________________________

____

10. List three methods of administering nitrates and nitrites.

a) ______________________________

____

b) ______________________________

____

c) ______________________________

____

11. List two categories of antianginal drugs other than the nitrates and an example of each category.

Categories	Drug Examples
a) ______________	a) ______________
b) ______________	b) ______________

12. Why is it necessary to treat hypertension? ______________________________

____

Define hypertension. ______________________________

____

Define secondary hypertension. ______________________________

____

13. What is the overall formula for blood pressure? ______

How do antihypertensive drugs alter factors that determine blood pressure? ______

14. Explain the mechanism a kidney uses to ensure adequate blood flow to the kidneys. ______

How does this mechanism affect hypertension? ______

15. Explain the "stair step" approach to the treatment of hypertension. ______

16. What are the three basic processes that occur in the formation of urine?

a) ______

b) ______

c) ______

Which of these processes is most important in the function of diurectics? ______

17. Explain the source hydrogen ions that are exchanged for sodium reabsorption in the kidney nephron.

18. Define the term diuretic. ______

What are the overall effects of diuretics? ______________________________

____

19. List the five classes of diuretics and explain the mechanism of action of each class. Also, give an example of a drug from each class.

Classes of Diuretics:	Mechanisms of Action:	Examples:
a) ______________	a) ______________	a) ______________
b) ______________	b) ______________	b) ______________
c) ______________	c) ______________	c) ______________
d) ______________	d) ______________	d) ______________

20. Other than diuretics, list four other categories of antihypertensive drugs with an example of a drug from each category.

Categories:	Drugs:
a) ______________	a) ______________
b) ______________	b) ______________
c) ______________	c) ______________
d) ______________	d) ______________

21. List the three end products of the coagulation process.

a) ______________________________

b) ______________________________

c) ______________________________

22. What are the two main categories of anticoagulant drugs?

a) ______________________________

b)______________________________

List three diseases for which these drugs are used.

a)______________________________

b)______________________________

c)______________________________

23. Compare heparin and the oral anticoagulants in terms of their mechanism of action, route of administration, antagonist, and drug interaction.

heparin:

a) mechanism of action: ______________________________

____

b) route of administration: ______________________________

____

c) antagonist: ______________________________

____

d) drug interaction: ______________________________

____

oral anticoagulants:

a) mechanism of action: ______________________________

____

b) route of administration: ______________________________

____

c) antagonist: ______________________________

____

d) drug interaction: ______________________________

____

24. Describe the importance of proper diet in controlling hyperlipidemia. ______________________________

____

List three important drugs used in the treatment of hyperlipidemia.

a) ______________________________

b) ______________________________

c) ______________________________

CHAPTER 6

Pharmacology of the Gastrointestinal Tract

Answer the following questions in your own words. Write your answers in the spaces provided.

1. Summarize the overall process of digestion. ______________________________

____

How does mucus protect the gastric lining from hydropic acid? ______________________________

____

2. Describe the two factors responsible for normal balance of GI function.

a) attack factors: ______________________________

____

____

b) resistance and defense factors: ______________________________

____

____

3. List five factors responsible for an increase in the incidence of ulcer disease or influence a balance between attack factors and resistance factors.

a) ______________________________

b) ______________________________

c) ______________________________

d) ______________________________

e) ______________________________

4. List three nonmedicinal factors that can decrease ulcer disease.

a) ______________________________

b) ______________________________

c) ______________________________

5. List two broad categories of drugs used in the treatment of ulcers.

a) ______________________________

b) ______________________________

6. Describe four groups of drugs that decrease attack factors. Give one example of each group.

Groups:	Examples:
a) ______________________ ______________________	a) ______________________
b) ______________________ ______________________	b) ______________________
c) ______________________ ______________________	c) ______________________
d) ______________________ ______________________	d) ______________________

7. Describe the mechanisms of action of the H_2 blockers and the proton pump inhibitor.

a) H_2 blockers: ______________________

____

b) proton pump inhibitor: ______________________

____

8. Describe the overall effect of the group of drugs that increases defense factors. ______________________

____

List two examples of these drugs.

a) ______________________

b) ______________________

9. Define and describe the following terms.

a) diarrhea: ______________________

____

____

b) constipation: ______________________

____

____

10. List three causes of diarrhea.

a) ______________________

b) ______________________

c) ______________________

What are the major problems associated with any type of diarrhea? ______________________

____

____

11. List four categories of antidiarrheal drugs. Give two examples of each category.

Categories:	Examples:
a) ______________	1) ______________
	2) ______________
b) ______________	1) ______________
	2) ______________
c) ______________	1) ______________
	2) ______________
d) ______________	1) ______________
	2) ______________

12. Define constipation. ______________________________

____

What causes constipation? ______________________________

____

13. Define the following terms.

a) laxative: ______________________________

b) cathartic: ______________________________

14. List four categories of laxative and cathartic drugs. Give an example of each category.

Categories:	Examples:
a) ______________	a) ______________
b) ______________	b) ______________
c) ______________	c) ______________
d) ______________	d) ______________

CHAPTER 7

Pharmacology of the Endocrine System

Answer the following questions in your own words. Write your answers in the spaces provided.

1. Explain how the hypothalamus controls the secretion of hormones from the adenohypophysis.

2. Explain how the hypothalamus controls the secretion of hormones from the neurohypophysis.

3. Define the term negative feedback.

Why does the word *negative* not have a bad connotation?

4. List three categories of corticosteroids secreted by the adrenal cortex.

a) ______________________________

b) ______________________________

c) ______________________________

Describe the function of each category of corticoids.

a) ______________________________

____

b) ______________________________

____

c) ______________________________

____

5. Describe the main therapeutic use of the glucocorticoids. ______________________________

____

____

What are the long-term side effects?

a) ______________________________

b) ______________________________

c) ______________________________

d) ______________________________

e) ______________________________

f) ______________________________

g) ______________________________

6. List three examples of synthetic glucocorticoids.

a) ______________________________

b) ______________________________

c) ______________________________

What advantage do synthetic glucocorticoids have over natural occurring glucocorticoids?

____

____

What are the side effects of synthetic glucocorticoids? ______

______

______

7. List the overall effects of the mineralocorticoids. ______

______

______

Name two examples of these agents.

a) ______

b) ______

8. Describe the overall effects of thyroxin. ______

______

______

Compare hypothyroidism to hyperthyroidism.

hypothyroidism: ______

______

______

hyperthyroidism: ______

______

______

9. Describe the treatment of hypothyroidism. ______

______

______

Give three examples of drugs used to treat hypothyroidism.

a) ______

b) ______

c) ______

10. Describe three approaches to the treatment of hyperthyroidism.

a) ______

b) ______

c) ______

List three examples of drugs to treat hyperthyroidism.

a) ______________________________

b) ______________________________

c) ______________________________

11. List the two hormones that control blood calcium and indicate the effects of each hormone on calcium levels.

a) ______________________________

b) ______________________________

12. Compare the effects of glucagon and insulin on blood glucose levels.

effects of glucagon: ______________________________

____

____

effects of insulin: ______________________________

____

____

13. Describe the main characteristics of diabetes mellitus and the causes of the characteristics.

Characteristics:	Causes:
a) ______________	a) ______________
b) ______________	b) ______________
c) ______________	c) ______________
d) ______________	d) ______________

e) ______________________ e) ______________________

____

____

f) ______________________ f) ______________________

____

____

g) ______________________ g) ______________________

____

____

14. Describe the overall treatment of diabetes mellitus. ______________________

____

____

Which drugs are used in the treatment of Type I diabetes? ______________________

____

____

Which drugs are used in the treatment of Type II diabetes? ______________________

____

____

15. Describe the overall physiological effects of histamine. ______________________

____

____

Compare the location of H1 and H2 receptor sites in the body.

a) vascular: ______________________

____

____

b) nonvascular: ______________________

____

____

c) heart effects: ______________________________

____

____

16. Describe why antihistamines are not effective in treating an acute anaphylactic allergic reaction.

____

____

____

____

17. List three commonly used antihistamine drugs.

a) ______________________________

b) ______________________________

c) ______________________________

Describe the most common side effects of antihistamine drugs.

a) ______________________________

b) ______________________________

c) ______________________________

How can these side effects be used therapeutically? ______________________________

____

____

CHAPTER 8

Antimicrobial Pharmacology

Answer the following questions in your own words. Write your answers in the spaces provided.

1. Compare the two methods by which antibiotics affect bacteria.

bacteriostatic: ____

____

____

bacteriocidal: ____

____

____

2. Define the term bacterial spectrum. ____

____

____

Differentiate between narrow and broad spectrum.

narrow spectrum: ____

____

____

broad spectrum: ____

____

____

3. Explain why it is important to use vigorous antibacterial therapy and avoid trivial use of antibiotics.

____

____

____

____

____

____

4. List five reasons for failure of antibacterial therapy.

a) ______________________________

____

b) ______________________________

____

c) ______________________________

____

d) ______________________________

____

e) ______________________________

____

5. Describe the basic mechanism of action of the beta-lactam antibiotics. Relate this action to chemical structures of the cell wall.

____

____

____

6. List at least one example of each of the four categories of the beta-lactam antibiotics.

a) Penicillins: ______________________________

b) Cephalosparus: ______________________________

c) Carbapenims: ______________________________

d) Monobatam: ______________________________

7. What is the significance in the incidence of allergies to beta-lactam antibiotics?

____

____

____

8. Explain the role of beta-lactamase inhibitors. ______________________________

____

____

Give an example of two antibiotics that have beta-lactam inhibitors added.

a) ______________________________

____

b) ______________________________

____

9. List an example of each of the three generations of cephalosporins.

first generation: ______________________________

second generation: ______________________________

third generation: ______________________________

10. Describe the main clinical use of erythromycin and vancomycin.

erythromycin: ______________________________

____

vancomycin: ______________________________

____

11. What is the main clinical adverse effect associated with aminoglycosides?

____

____

____

12. What is meant by broad spectrum? ______________________________

____

What is the use of choramphenicol? ______________________________

____

13. Why is it important to avoid taking tetracycline with calcium products? ______________________________

____

____

Why should tetracyclines *not* be given to children under the age of 12? ______________________________

____

____

14. Describe the mechanism of sulfonamides. ______________________________

____

____

What are today's main clinicals uses of sulfonamides? ______________________________

____

____

15. List two categories of fungal infections and an example of one antifungal drug used in the treatment of each category.

Categories:	Examples:
a) ______________	a) ______________
b) ______________	b) ______________

16. Describe two approaches to the treatment of viral diseases.

a) ______________________________

b) ______________________________

What are the main clinical uses of acyclovir and ribavirin?

acyclovir: ______________________________

____

____

ribavirin: ______________________________

____

____

CHAPTER 9

Pharmacology of Chemotherapy

Answer the following questions in your own words. Write your answers in the spaces provided.

1. Explain two characteristics of cancer cells.

   a) ______________________________

   b) ______________________________

   Describe the following terms.

   a) malignant: ______________________________

   ____

   b) benign: ______________________________

   ____

2. List three approaches to cancer treatment. Indicate the effectiveness and rationale for each approach.

   a) ______________________________

   ____

   b) ______________________________

   ____

   c) ______________________________

   ____

3. What is the rationale behind the use of chemotherapy on cancer? ______________________________

   ____

   ____

   Why are chemotherapuetic agents so toxic? ______________________________

   ____

   ____

4. List two main categories of chemotherapeutic drugs.

a) ______________________________

b) ______________________________

What are the mechanisms of action of the above categories?

a) ______________________________

b) ______________________________

5. List three categories of miscellaneous anticancer drugs. Give one example of each.

Categories:	Examples:
a) ______________	a) ______________
b) ______________	b) ______________
c) ______________	c) ______________

Describe the function of these devices when used with MDI therapy. ______

______

______

______

______

______

7. Define drug administration by instillation. ______

______

______

______

Describe three indications for instillation of drugs.

a) ______

______

b) ______

______

c) ______

______

8. Describe the disadvantages and hazards of drug administration by instillation.

Disadvantages: ______

______

______

______

______

Hazards: ______

______

______

______

______

CHAPTER 11

Bronchodilator Therapy

Answer the following questions in your own words. Write your answers in the spaces provided.

1. Define bronchoconstriction. ______________________________

____

____

____

____

2. There are three mechanisms (causes) of bronchoconstriction. Bronchoconstriction may be caused by:

   a) ______________________________

   ____

   b) ______________________________

   ____

   c) ______________________________

   ____

3. Why is it important to identify the cause of bronchoconstriction? ______________________________

____

____

____

4. Describe appropriate respiratory care for the reversal of bronchoconstriction caused by excess or retained secretions.

____

____

____

____

____

____

5. Describe appropriate respiratory care for the reversal of bronchoconstriction caused by mucosal edema.

6. Describe appropriate respiratory care for the reversal of bronchoconstriction caused by bronchospasm.

7. Describe the reaction within a bronchial smooth muscle cell when a β_2 receptor is stimulated.

8. What is cyclic 3'5'-adenosine monophophosphate (cAMP)?

What is its role in the relief of bronchospasms?

9. What is phosphodiesterase? ______________________________

____

____

How does it effect cAMP? ______________________________

____

____

10. What is the effect of cholinergic stimulation of a bronchial smooth muscle cell? ______________

____

____

11. There are three categories of bronchodilators, defined by their mechanisms of action. These three categories are:

a) ______________________________

b) ______________________________

c) ______________________________

12. Define the term sympathomimetic. ______________________________

____

____

What term is often used as a synonym for sympathomimetic? ______________

____

____

13. Describe how sympathomimetic bronchodilators achieve relief of bronchospasm. (Hint: What is the mechanism of action?)

____

____

____

____

____

____

____

____

14. Draw a diagram showing the chemical mediators and reactions that occur when a sympathomimetic (β-adrenergic) bronchodilator is given.

15. Define the term anticholinergic.________________________

What term can be used as a synonym for anticholinergic? ________________________

16. Described how parasympatholytic bronchodilators achieve relief of bronchospasm. ________________________

What is the mechanism of action? ________________________

Six sympathomimetic bronchodilators are listed in problems 17 through 22. Fill in the blanks for each bronchodilator.

17. Albuterol

a) Brand names: ________________________

b) Alpha and beta effects: ______________________________

____

c) Dosage (in volume and weight) and frequency (include the concentration of each solution):

____

____

____

d) Duration of effectiveness: ______________________________

e) Contraindications: ______________________________

____

____

____

f) Side effects: ______________________________

____

____

____

g) Special considerations (if any): ______________________________

____

____

____

____

18. Isoetharine

a) Brand names: ______________________________

b) Alpha and beta effects: ______________________________

____

c) Dosage (in volume and weight) and frequency (include the concentration of each solution):

____

____

____

d) Duration of effectiveness: ______

e) Contraindications: ______

______

______

______

f) Side effects: ______

______

______

______

g) Special considerations (if any): ______

______

______

______

______

19. Isoproterenol

a) Brand names: ______

______

______

b) Alpha and beta effects: ______

______

c) Dosage (in volume and weight) and frequency (include the concentration of each solution):

______

______

______

______

d) Duration of effectiveness: ______

e) Contraindications: ______

______

______

______

f) Side effects: ____________________

____

____

____

g) Special considerations (if any): ____________________

____

____

____

____

20. Metaproterenol

a) Brand names: ____________________

____

b) Alpha and beta effects: ____________________

____

c) Dosage (in volume and weight) and frequency (include the concentration of each solution):

____

____

____

____

d) Duration of effectiveness: ____________________

e) Contraindications: ____________________

____

____

____

f) Side effects: ____________________

____

____

____

g) Special considerations (if any): ______

______

______

______

______

21. Racemic epinephrine

a) Brand names: ______

______

______

b) Alpha and beta effects: ______

______

c) Dosage (in volume and weight) and frequency (include the concentration of each solution):

______

______

______

______

d) Duration of effectiveness: ______

e) Contraindications: ______

______

______

______

f) Side effects: ______

______

______

______

g) Special considerations (if any): ______

______

______

______

______

22. Terbutaline

a) Brand names: ____________________

____

b) Alpha and beta effects: ____________________

____

c) Dosage (in volume and weight) and frequency (include the concentration of each solution):

____

____

____

____

d) Duration of effectiveness: ____________________

e) Contraindications: ____________________

____

____

____

f) Side effects: ____________________

____

____

____

g) Special considerations (if any): ____________________

____

____

____

____

23. List two potent, long acting, β_2 -specific bronchodilators currently available only in MDI.

____

____

There are two anticholinergic bronchodilators currently in use. Fill in the blanks of the following.

24. Atropine sulfate

a) Dosage and frequency:____________________

b) Duration of effectiveness: ____________________

c) Contraindications:____________________

d) Side effects: ____________________

e) Special considerations (if any): ____________________

25. Ipratropium bromide

a) Brand names: ____________________

b) Dosage and frequency:____________________

c) Duration of effectiveness: ____________________

c) Contraindications: ______

d) Side effects: ______

e) Special considerations (if any): ______

26. Describe the use of xanthines in the control of bronchospasms. ______

27. Describe how xanthines achieve relief of bronchospasm. ______

What is the mechanism of action? ______

28. Why would a patient be receiving both ipratropium and albuterol for control of bronchospasms?

______

CHAPTER 12

Wetting Agents and Mucolytics

Answer the following questions in your own words. Write your answers in the spaces provided.

1. Define the following terms.

a) bland aerosol: ____

____

____

____

b) wetting agents: ____

____

____

____

c) mucolysis: ____

____

d) mucolytic: ____

____

____

e) hygroscopic: ____

____

____

f) expectorant: ____

____

____

g) bronchorrhea: ____

____

2. List three bland aerosols.

a) ______

b) ______

c) ______

3. Describe the patient-care situations in which:

a) normal saline would be preferable to sterile distilled water as a wetting agent. ______

______

______

______

b) half-normal saline would be preferable to normal saline. ______

______

______

______

c) sterile water would be preferable to normal saline. ______

______

______

______

4. Describe the composition of a normal mucus molecule. ______

______

______

______

5. List three types (categories) of mucolytics.

a) ______

b) ______

c) ______

6. Describe how *N*-acetylcysteine accomplishes mucolysis. ______________________________

7. Describe how aerosolized sodium bicarbonate accomplishes mucolysis. ______________________________

8. List the contraindications for use of sodium bicarbonate as a mucolytic. ______________________________

9. List the contraindications for the use of *N*-acetylcysteine as a mucolytic. ______________________________

10. List the hazards or side effects of *N*-acteylcysteine when used as a mucolytic. ______________________________

11. Define the concentrations and dosage ranges for sodium bicarbonate as a mucolytic.

Concentration(s): ______________________________

Dosage(s): ______________________________

12. Define the concentrations and dosage ranges for *N*-acetylcysteine as a mucolytic.

Concentration(s): ______________________________

Dosage(s): ______________________________

13. Describe a patient-care situation in which *N*-acetylcysteine may be ordered for a nonrespiratory diagnosis.

____

____

14. Define sputum induction. ____

____

Which wetting agent would be appropriate for this use? ____

____

15. What is the most effective approach for maintaining normal pulmonary secretions and their mobilization?

____

____

CHAPTER 13

Aerosol Antimicrobial Therapy

Answer the following questions in your own words. Write your answers in the spaces provided.

1. List six indications for the use of antimicrobial drugs by aerosol administration.

   a) ______

   b) ______

   c) ______

   d) ______

   e) ______

   f) ______

2. List ten disadvantages or limitations of delivering antimicrobial drugs by aerosol route.

   a) ______

   b) ______

   c) ______

   d) ______

   e) ______

   f) ______

   g) ______

   h) ______

   i) ______

   j) ______

3. What is the most common adverse reaction to the administration of aerosolized antimicrobials? ______

   ______

4. Describe three specific pulmonary infectious processes that have been successfully and appropriately treated by the use of aerosolized antimicrobials.

   a) ______

   ______

b) ____________________

____

c) ____________________

____

5. List four categories of antimicrobial drugs that may be given by aerosol.

a) ____________________

b) ____________________

c) ____________________

d) ____________________

Six antibacterial drugs that have been used successfully by aerosol route are listed in problems 6 through 11. Fill in the blanks following each drug.

6. Amoxicillin

a) Brand names: ____________________

____

____

____

b) Clinical indications (i.e., spectrum and specific diseases/conditions for which it has been used):

____

____

____

c) Contraindications: ____________________

____

d) Adverse reactions or side effects: ____________________

____

____

e) Dosage: ____________________

____

____

f) Special considerations (if any): ______________________________

____

____

____

7. Carbenicillin

a) Brand names: ______________________________

____

____

b) Clinical indications (i.e., spectrum and specific diseases/conditions for which it has been used):

____

____

____

c) Contraindications: ______________________________

____

d) Adverse reactions or side effects: ______________________________

____

____

e) Dosage: ______________________________

____

____

f) Special considerations (if any): ______________________________

____

____

____

8. Colistin

a) Brand names: ______________________________

____

b) Clinical indications (i.e., spectrum and specific diseases/conditions for which it has been used):

____

____

____

c) Contraindications: ______________________________

____

d) Adverse reactions or side effects: ______________________________

____

____

e) Dosage: ______________________________

____

____

f) Special considerations (if any): ______________________________

____

____

____

9. Gentamincin

a) Brand names: ______________________________

____

b) Clinical indications (i.e., spectrum and specific diseases/conditions for which it has been used):

____

____

____

c) Contraindications: ______________________________

____

d) Adverse reactions or side effects: ______________________________

____

____

e) Dosage: ______________________________

____

____

f) Special considerations (if any): ______________________________

____

____

____

10. Kanamycin

a) Brand names: ______________________________

____

b) Clinical indications (i.e., spectrum and specific diseases/conditions for which it has been used):

____

____

____

c) Contraindications: ______________________________

____

d) Adverse reactions or side effects: ______________________________

____

____

e) Dosage: ______________________________

____

____

f) Special considerations (if any): ____________________

____

____

____

11. Polymixin B

a) Brand name: ____________________

b) Clinical indications (i.e., spectrum and specific diseases/conditions for which it has been used):

____

____

____

c) Contraindications: ____________________

____

d) Adverse reactions or side effects: ____________________

____

____

e) Dosage: ____________________

____

____

f) Special considerations (if any): ____________________

____

____

____

Two antifungal drugs have been used successfully by aerosol route. For each drug in problems 12 and 13, fill in the blanks.

12. Amphotericin B

a) Brand name: ____________________

b) Clinical indications (i.e., spectrum and specific diseases/conditions for which it has been used):

c) Contraindications:

d) Adverse reactions or side effects:

e) Dosage:

f) Special considerations (if any):

13. Nystatin

a) Brand name:

b) Clinical indications (i.e., spectrum and specific diseases/conditions for which it has been used):

c) Contraindications:

d) Adverse reactions or side effects:

e) Dosage: ______________________________

____

____

f) Special considerations (if any): ______________________________

____

____

____

14. Describe the one antiviral drug that has been successfully used by aerosol route-ribavirin.

a) Brand name: ______________________________

b) Clinical indications (i.e., spectrum and specific diseases/conditions for which it has been used):

____

____

____

c) Contraindications: ______________________________

____

d) Adverse reactions or side effects: ______________________________

____

____

e) Dosage: ______________________________

____

____

f) Special considerations (if any): ______________________________

____

____

____

15. What is an SPAG nebulizer? ______

When is its use indicated (or required)? ______

16. Describe the antiprotozoal drug that has been successfully given by aerosol route-pentamidine.

a) Brand names: ______

b) Clinical indications (i.e., spectrum and specific diseases/conditions for which it has been used):

c) Contraindications: ______

d) Adverse reactions or side effects: ______

e) Dosage: ______

f) Special considerations (if any): ______________________________

____

____

____

17. Why should the respiratory care practitioner be knowledgeable regarding rare applications, such as the use of aerosolized antimicrobials?

____

____

____

18. What actions should be taken if there is a question regarding the FDA-approved status of aerosolizing a specific antimicrobial?

____

____

____

CHAPTER 14

Anti-Inflammatory and Antiasthmatic Drugs

Answer the following questions in your own words. Write your answers in the spaces provided.

1. Define the term mucosal edema. ______

______

______

2. List several diseases or conditions that may cause mucosal edema from the following etiologies.

   a) infectious processes: ______

   ______

   ______

   b) inhalation injury: ______

   ______

   ______

   c) airway trauma: ______

   ______

   d) diseases: ______

   ______

   e) conditions: ______

   ______

3. Describe how an α-adrenergic drug reduces mucosal edema. ______

______

______

Two α-adrenergic drugs are used by respiratory care practitioners. Describe each of the drugs in problems 4 and 5 by filling in the blanks.

4. Epinephrine

   a) Brand names: ______

   ______

   ______

   ______

   ______

b) Dosage and frequency: ______________________________

____

____

____

____

c) Duration of effectiveness: ______________________________

d) Contraindications: ______________________________

____

____

e) Side effects: ______________________________

____

____

f) Special considerations (if any): ______________________________

____

____

____

____

____

____

5. Racemic epinephrine

a) Brand names: ______________________________

____

____

b) Dosage and frequency: ______________________________

____

____

____

____

c) Duration of effectiveness: ______________________________

d) Contraindications: ______________________________

e) Side effects: ______

______

______

f) Special considerations (if any): ______

______

______

______

______

6. Describe the mechanism of action of corticosteroids. ______

______

______

______

______

7. Describe the rationale for the use of aerosolized corticosteroids. ______

______

______

What are the two advantages of aerosol administration as compared to oral administration? ______

a) ______

b) ______

8. What are four disadvantages of aerosolized corticosteriods? ______

a) ______

b) ______

c) ______

d) ______

9. What special precautions should be taken when initiating aerosol corticosteroid therapy? ______

______

______

______

______

What specific patient education should occur to ensure safe and effective aerosol corticosteroid therapy?

____

____

____

____

10. What are four potential side effects or adverse reactions of aerosolized corticosteriods?

a) _______________

b) _______________

c) _______________

d) _______________

Four corticosteroids currently used by aerosol route are listed in problems 11 through 14. Fill in the blanks for each drug.

11. Beclomethasone

a) Brand names: _______________

____

b) Duration: _______________

____

c) Dosage: _______________

____

____

____

d) Special considerations (if any): _______________

____

____

____

12. Dexamethasone

a) Brand name: _______________

b) Duration: _______________

____

c) Dosage: ______________________________

____

____

____

d) Special considerations (if any): ______________________________

____

____

____

13. Flunisolide

a) Brand name: ______________________________

b) Duration: ______________________________

____

c) Dosage: ______________________________

____

____

____

d) Special considerations (if any): ______________________________

____

____

____

14. Triamcinolone

a) Brand name: ______________________________

b) Duration: ______________________________

____

c) Dosage: ______________________________

____

____

____

d) Special considerations (if any): ________________

____

____

____

15. Describe the role of the mast cell in the allergic response. ________________

____

____

____

16. Describe the mechanism of action in cromolyn sodium. ________________

____

____

____

17. Describe the indications, contraindications, limitations, and concerns for the use of cromolyn sodium.

Indications: ________________

____

Contraindications: ________________

____

____

____

Limitations: ________________

____

____

Concerns: ________________

____

18. Describe cromolyn sodium, including

a) Brand name: ________________

____

b) Duration: ________________

____

c) Dosage and frequency: ______

d) Adverse reactions/side effects: ______

e) Special considerations (if any): ______

19. Describe the Spinhaler and its use (and limitations) in cromolyn sodium therapy.

______

20. Describe the mechanism of action in nedocromil sodium. ______

21. Describe the indications, contraindications, limitations, and concerns fo the use of nedocromil sodium.

Indications: ____________________

____

____

____

Contraindications: ____________________

____

____

____

Limitations: ____________________

____

____

Concerns: ____________________

____

22. Describe nedocromil sodium, including

a) Brand name: ____________________

b) Duration: ____________________

____

____

c) Dosage and frequency: ____________________

____

____

____

d) Adverse reactions/side effects: ____________________

____

____

____

____

23. A newly-diagnosed asthmatic is placed on a treatment regimen of albuterol, Asmacort®, and Intal®. The patient seems skeptical about the need for "so many drugs." As a practitioner, you are concerned about the patient's compliance with drug therapy after being discharged. How would you explain how each drug is different and why they are all needed? Explain whether or not there is a specific sequence in which the drugs should be taken.

24. You are called to the ER on a Saturday night to treat an asthmatic in acute distress. The physician has ordered an immediate treatment of 20 mg cromolyn sodium and blood gases. No other therapy has been ordered. What is your reaction? How could you advise the physician?

CHAPTER 15

Surface Active Agents

Answer the following questions in your own words. Write your answers in the spaces provided.

1. Define the term surface tension. __________

2. Describe how surface tension effects the work of breathing, particularly in the newborn.

3. Define the following terms.

   a) surfactant (general terms): __________

   b) pulmonary surfactant: __________

4. Describe the indications for the use of surfactant-replacement drugs, including both prevention and rescue protocols.

____

____

____

____

____

____

____

There are two surfactant-replacement drugs currently in use in the United States. Describe each of the drugs in problems 5 and 6.

5. Beractant

a) Brand name: ______________________________

b) Indications/prevention protocol: ______________________________

____

____

Indications/rescue protocol: ______________________________

____

____

c) Contraindications: ______________________________

d) Dosage and route of administration: ______________________________

____

____

____

____

e) Adverse reactions/side effects: ______________________________

____

____

____

____

f) Special considerations (if any): ____________________

____

____

____

____

6. Colfosceril palmitate, cetyl alcohol, tyloxapol

a) Brand name: ____________________

b) Indications/prevention protocol: ____________________

____

____

Indications/rescue protocol: ____________________

____

____

c) Contraindications: ____________________

d) Dosage and route of administration: ____________________

____

____

____

____

e) Adverse reactions/side effects: ____________________

____

____

____

____

f) Special considerations (if any): ____________________

____

____

____

____

7. Define the following terms.

interstitial pulmonary edema: ______________________________

fulminant pulmonary edema: ______________________________

alveolar pulmonary edema: ______________________________

8. List the predisposing or causative factors that may lead to the development of fulminant alveolar pulmonary edema.

____

9. Describe the clinical signs and symptoms associated with fulminant alveolar pulmonary edema.

Vital signs: ______________________________

Level of consciousness: ______________________________

Blood gases/oxygenation: ______________________________

Breath sounds: ____

____

Chest radiograph findings: ____

____

____

10. Describe the mechanism of action by which ethyl alcohol reduces the secretions associated with alveolar pulmonary edema.

____

____

____

____

____

____

____

11. Describe the dosage concentration and frequency of aerosol administration of ethyl alcohol for the treatment of alveolar pulmonary edema. List any special considerations also.

Dosage/concentration: ____

____

____

Frequency: ____

Special considerations: ____

____

____

____

____

CHAPTER 16

Special Applications

Answer the following questions in your own words. Write your answers in the spaces provided.

1. How are infants and children defined, for the purposes of determining drug doses?

infants: ______________________________

____

____

children: ______________________________

____

____

____

2. Approximately what percentage of currently FDA-approved drugs specify "safe and effective" pediatric dosages?

____

____

3. Define the term titration as it applies to adjusting infant and pediatric drug dosages. ______________

____

____

____

____

4. There are three generally accepted rules for determining an appropriate initial drug dosage for children over the age of two. For each rule, calculate the initial dosage of Ventolin® to be given to an eight-year-old child who weighs 60 pounds. (Hint: Write each rule and then calculate dosage.)

a) Clark's Rule: ______________________________

____

____

____

Dosage: ______________________________

____

____

____

b) Cowling's Rule: ______________________________

____

____

____

Dosage: ______________________________

____

____

____

c) Young's Rule: ______________________________

____

____

____

Dosage: ______________________________

____

____

____

5. How do the calculated initial dosages recommended by each rule compare? ______________________________

____

____

6. How should drug dosage be determined *after* the initial treatment is given with a "recommended" dosage?

____

____

____

7. Fried's Rule applies to children under the age of two. Use this rule to calculate an *initial* dosage of Proventil® for a child in the ER who is 18 months old and weighs 22 pounds.

Fried's Rule: ______________________________

____

____

____

Dosage: ______________________________

____

____

____

8. What organizations publish guidelines for determining drug dosages for infants and children? ______________

____

____

9. According to the 1992 DHHS report, *Executive Summary: Guidelines for the Diagnosis and Management of Asthma,* what are the recommended pediatric dosages for the following drugs?

albuterol: ______________________________

____

maximum pediatric dose: ______________________________

metaproterenol: ______________________________

____

maximum pediatric dose: ______________________________

beclomethasone: ______________________________

cromolyn sodium: ______________________________

____

10. What is ACLS? ______________________________

What general content areas are included in an ACLS course?

a) ______________________________

b) ______________________________

c) ______________________________

d) ______________________________

e) ______________________________

f) ______________________________

g) ______________________________

h) ______________________________

i) ______________________________

j) ______________________________

k) ______________________________

11. Where is your local affiliate of the American Heart Association? ______________________________

____

Where is ACLS training available? ______________________________

____

What entry-criteria is necessary for ACLS training? ______________________________

____

12. For each drug included in cardiac resuscitation and advanced cardiac life support (as defined by American Heart Association protocol), describe the drug category (action). List brand name(s):

drug name: epinephrine

actions: ______________________________

____

____

____

Why is this drug used for cardiac resuscitation/care? ______________________________

____

____

____

drug name: atropine

actions: ______________________________

____

____

____

____

Why is this drug used for cardiac resuscitation/care? ______________________________

____

____

____

drug name: lidocaine

brand name(s): ______

actions: ______

______

______

______

______

______

Why is this drug used for cardiac resuscitation/care? ______

______

______

______

drug name: procainamide

brand name(s): ______

actions: ______

______

______

______

______

______

Why is this drug used for cardiac resuscitation/care? ______

______

______

______

drug name: bretylium

brand name(s): ______

actions: ______

______

______

______

______

Why is this drug used for cardiac resuscitation/care? ______________________________

____

____

____

drug name: verapamil

brand name(s): ______________________________

actions: ______________________________

____

____

____

____

____

Why is this drug used for cardiac resuscitation/care? ______________________________

____

____

____

drug name: morphine

brand name(s): ______________________________

actions: ______________________________

____

____

____

____

____

Why is this drug used for cardiac resuscitation/care? ______________________________

____

____

____

drug name: sodium bicarbonate

brand name(s): ______

actions: ______

Why is this drug used for cardiac resuscitation/care? ______

drug name: norepinephrine

actions: ______

Why is this drug used for cardiac resuscitation/care? ______

drug name: dopamine

brand name(s): ______

actions: ______

Why is this drug used for cardiac resuscitation/care? ____________________

____

____

____

drug name: dobutamine

brand name(s): ____________________

actions: ____________________

____

____

____

____

____

Why is this drug used for cardiac resuscitation/care? ____________________

____

____

____

drug name: isoproterenol

brand name(s): ____________________

actions: ____________________

____

____

____

____

____

Why is this drug used for cardiac resuscitation/care? ____________________

____

____

____

drug name: digitalis

brand name(s): ____________________

actions: ____________________

Why is this drug used for cardiac resuscitation/care? ____________________

drug name: sodium nitroprusside

brand name(s): ____________________

actions: ____________________

Why is this drug used for cardiac resuscitation/care? ____________________

drug name: nitroglycerin

brand name(s): ____________________

actions: ____________________

Why is this drug used for cardiac resuscitation/care? ______________________________

drug name: propranolol

brand name(s): ______________________________

actions: ______________________________

Why is this drug used for cardiac resuscitation/care? ______________________________

drug name: furosemide

brand name(s): ______________________________

actions: ______________________________

Why is this drug used for cardiac resuscitation/care? ______________________________

13. What protocols have been established for the use of the ACLS drugs? ______

Where are these protocols published? ______

14. What special considerations should be observed by the respiratory care practitioner when assisting a physician with a bronchoscopy? (Describe patient assessment and monitoring, as well as equipment that should be available.)

15. Describe the use of lidocaine as indicated for use before or during bronchoscopy.

16. Define the following regarding lidocaine when used before or during bronchoscopy.

a) brand name: ______________________________

____

____

b) actions: ______________________________

____

____

c) duration: ______________________________

d) contraindications: ______________________________

____

e) dosage/pre-procedure aerosol: ______________________________

____

dosage/mid-procedure instillation: ______________________________

____

17. Describe the drug methacholine.

brand name (s): ______________________________

actions: ______________________________

____

What is the procedure during which methacholine is used? ______________________________

____

18. Describe the appropriate use of methacholine as a diagnostic agent, including any special considerations that should be observed by the RCP when using this drug.

contraindications to methacholine administration: ______________________________

____

____

dosage: ______________________________

____

special equipment/precautions: ______________________________

____

Dosage Calculation Problems

Complete the following dosage calculations. Write your answers in the spaces provided.

1. How much racemic epinephrine does a patient receive if the treatment is given with 0.25 ml Vaponefrin®? (Hint: What is the solution strength of Vaponefrin®? Calculate how many milligrams of racemic epinephrine are present in each ml of solution.)

answer:____________________

2. How much albuterol does a patient receive if the treatment is given with 0.30 ml Proventil®? (Hint: What is the solution strength of Proventil®? Calculate how many milligrams of albuterol are present in each ml of solution.

answer:____________________

3. How much isoetharine does the patient receive if the treatment is given with 0.50 ml Bronkosol®? (Hint: What is the solution strength of Bronkosol®? Calculate how many milligrams of isoetharine are present in each ml of solution.)

answer:____________________

4. How much isoproterenol does the patient receive if the treatment is given with 0.50 ml of a 1:100 solution of Isuprel®? (Hint: What is the concentration of a 1:100 solution? Calculate how many milligrams of isoproterenol are present in each ml of solution.)

answer:________________________

5. How much metaproterenol does the patient receive if the treatment is given with 0.40 ml Alupent®? (Hint: What is the solution strength of Alupent®? Calculate how many milligrams of metaproterenol are present in each ml of solution.)

answer:________________________

6. How many ampules of 0.1% terbutaline must be used for a treatment order of 1.50 mg? (Hint: Calculate how many milligrams of terbutaline are present in each ml of solution.)

answer:________________________

7. How much Isuprel® 1:200 must be given if a patient in status asthmaticus has an order to receive 2.50 mg of isoproterenol diluted with 1.50 ml normal saline? (Hint: What is the concentration of a 1:200 solution? Calculate how many milligrams of isoproterenol are present in each ml of solution.)

answer: ______________________

8. How much Racepinephrine® must be given to satisfy a physician's order for an aerosol treatment with 10 mg racemic epinephrine in 2.50 ml normal saline? (Hint: What is the solution strength of Racepinephrine®? Calculate how many milligrams of racemic epinephrine are present in each ml of solution.)

answer: ______________________

9. How much Mucomyst® must be used to provide an aerosol of 3.0 ml of 10% *N*-acetylcysteine if the only available multiple-dose vials of Mucomyst® are 20% concentration?

answer: ______________________

Bonus: Should anything else be suggested in conjunction with the Mucomyst®?

____

10. How much Coly-Mycin S® must be given if a treatment is ordered with 100 mg of colistin? (Hint: Coly-Mycin S® is provided in 150 mg vials, which are reconstituted with 2.0 ml sterile water.)

answer: ______________________

11. How much ribavirin is delivered if 300 ml of a 2% solution are nebulized? (Hint: Calculate how many milligrams of ribavirin are present in each ml of solution.)

answer: ______________________

Bonus: What is the dosage per hour in the dose in problem 11 if nebulized over a 12-hour period?

____

Comprehensive Exam

1. Match the descriptions on the right to the appropriate principles of pharmacology on the left.

Absorption _________	a) the method of eliminating drugs from the body
Distribution _________	b) biotransformation
Metabolism _________	c) to pass through
Excretion _________	d) carrying a drug to a receptor site

2. Match the appropriate description from the list on the right to the list of factors that alter drug response on the left.

Patient compliance _________	a) presence of lung disease or kidney failure
Pathologic state _________	b) drug A effects the metabolism for drug B
Age of patient _________	c) failure to take a drug at the appropriate time
Drug interaction _________	d) liver is not fully functional in a child

3. The overall function of the autonomic nervous system controls all of the following except:

   a) the heart rate.

   b) the urinary bladder.

   c) glandular secretions.

   d) skeletal muscle.

4. All of the following statements about neurotransmitters are true except:

   a) Neurotransmitters are released at synaptic junctions.

   b) The neurotransmitters are at the neuroeffector site in the parasympathetic nervous system is acetylcholine.

   c) The neurotransmitter at the ganglion site in the sympathetic nervous system is N.E.

   d) The neurotransmitter at the neuromuscular junction in the somatic nervous system is acetylcholine.

5. Which category of sympathometic drugs is most important to a respiratory care practitioner?

   a) α-adrenergic

   b) β-blockers

   c) α-blockers

   d) β-adrenergic

   e) neuronal blockers

6. Which of the two categories of cholinergic drugs increases the activity of the parasympathetic system?

   a) anticholinesterase drugs

   b) anticholinergic drugs

7. The most important anticholinergic drug as far as clinical use by the RCP is:

   a) scopolamine.

   b) propantheline (Pro-Banthine®).

   c) atropine.

   d) tropicamide (Mydriacyl®).

8. All of the following characteristics of CNS drugs are true except:

   a) Acute or chronic excitation by a drug is often followed by a period of depression.

   b) Low doses of some depressant drugs can cause excitation.

   c) Chronic depression that is drug induced is followed by a period of excitation.

   d) Antagonist between stimulants and depressants is quite predictable.

   e) Many CNS drugs are addictive when administered together.

9. All of the following are clinical uses of barbiturates except:

   a) anticonvulsants.

   b) sedative/hypnotics.

   c) analgesia.

   d) antianxiety.

   e) induction of general anesthesia.

10. Match the appropriate drug from the list on the right, to the list of psychopharmacologic categories on the left.

Mood stabilizer _________	a) methyphenidate (Ritalin®)
Psychostimulant _________	b) imipramine (Tofranil®)
Antianxiety _________	c) chlorpromazine (Thorazine®)
Antidepressants _________	d) chlordiazepoxide (Librium®)
Antipsychotic _________	e) lithium carbonate

11. All of the following are effected by narcotic analgesics. Which system is the greatest concern for the RCP?

a) cardiovascular

b) central nervous system

c) GI tract

d) skin and its derivatives

e) hepatic system

12. Which of the following properties do acetaminophen (Tylenol®) and ibuprofen (Motrin®) *not* have in common?

a) antipyretic

b) analgesic

c) anti-inflammatory

d) anticoagulant

13. All of the following result in a decrease in flow in the coronary arteries except:

a) arthrosclerosis.

b) congestive heart failure.

c) angina pectoris.

d) myocardial infarction.

14. Match the mechanisms of action from the list on the right to the appropriate antiarrhythmic drug groups on the left.

Propranolol (Inderal®)__________	a) calcium channel blocker
Bretylium __________	b) β-blocker
Verapamil (Calan®) __________	c) sodium channel blocker
Procainamide (Pronestyl®) __________	d) adrenergic neuronal blocker

15. Diuretics are drugs used for all of the following pathological conditions except:

a) congestive heart failure.

b) hypertension.

c) glaucoma.

d) hypotension.

16. Which of the following diuretic categories causes the most profound diuresis?

a) loop diuretics

b) potassium sparing

c) thiazide

d) carbonic anhydrase inhibitors

e) osmotic

17. All of the following statements about anticoagulants are true except:

a) Heparin has an immediate onset of action.

b) An anticoagulant to warfarin is vitamin K.

c) Drug interactions are very common with the use of heparin.

d) Oral anticoagulants are monitored by the prothrobin time.

18. All of the following drugs are H_2 blockers except:

a) omeprazole (Prilosec®).

b) cimetidine (Tagamet®).

c) ranitidine (Zantac®).

d) famotidine (Pepcid®).

19. Match the steroid with its appropriate function on the right to the list of corticosteroids on the left.

Mineralocorticoid _________	a) has affect on the testes and ovaries
Glucocorticoids _________	b) controls sodium and potassium balance
Gonadocorticoid _________	c) increases glucose levels

20. All of the following statements about Type I and Type II diabetes are true except:

a) Type I and Type II can both be treated by diet alone.

b) Type I diabetes requires insulin.

c) Type II diabetes requires only oral hypoglycemic agents.

d) With both types diet is important.

21. All of the following are effects of histamine except:

a) decrease in blood pressure.

b) decrease in heart rate.

c) bronchiole constriction.

d) contraction of the small intestines.

22. Match the definitions in the list on the right to the list of terms on the left.

Antibiotic _________	a) inhibits growth
Antimicrobial _________	b) selectivity against a group of organisms
Bacteriostatic _________	c) kills or inhibits growth of any microorganism
Bacteriocidal _________	d) produced by living organisms
Spectrum _________	e) kills bacteria

23. Match the categories from the list on the right to the list of categories of penicillins on the left.

Natural penicillins _________	a) colaxacillin
Penicillinase resistant _________	b) amoxicillin
Amino penicillins _________	c) carbenicillin
Extended spectrum _________	d) penicillin G

24. Which one of the following drugs is effective against both anaerobic bacteria and parasitic infection, such as amebiasis and giardiasis?

a) streptomycin

b) clindamycin (Cleocin®)

c) metronidazole (Flagyl®)

d) norfloxacin (Noroxin®)

25. Which of the following sulfonamide drugs is currently used in treating ulcerative colitis?

a) silver sulfadiazine (Silvadene®)

b) sulfasalazine (Azulfidine®)

c) sulfacetamide (Sulamyd®)

d) trimethoprim-sulfamethoxazole (Septra®)

26. If early diagnosis of a cancer has not occurred, which one of the following treatments is most likely to be successful?

a) surgery

b) radiation

c) chemotherapy

d) combination of b and c

e) combination of a, b and c, if accessible

27. Which of the following solutions has a mucolytic effect?

I. hypotonic saline

II. isotonic saline

III. *N*-acetylcysteine 10%

IV. *N*-acetylcysteine 20%

V. sodium bicarbonate 4.2%

a) I, III, and IV only

b) II, III, IV, and V only

c) III only

d) III, IV and V only

e) I, II, IV, and V only

28. It is essential to use a bronchodilator in conjunction with which of the following mucolytics?

a) *N*-acetylcysteine 10%

b) SSKI

c) sodium bicarbonate 2.4%

c) hypotonic saline

e) all of the above

29. Which of the following drug categories is routinely administered by instillation?

a) bronchodilators, mucolytics, and drying agents

b) mucolytics, surfactant replacement drugs, and wetting agents

c) antibiotics, surfactant replacement drugs, and bronchodilators

d) ACLS drugs and mucolytics

e) none of the above are correct

30. Which of the following drugs is a β_2-specific bronchodilator?

a) Azmacort®

b) Atrovent®

c) albuterol

d) atropine

e) all of the above are β_2-specific

31. Which of the following sympathomimetic bronchodilators has the longest duration of effectiveness?

a) isoproterenol

b) isoetharine

c) metaproterenol

d) albuterol

e) pirbuterol

32. Which of the following clinical situations may justify the need for an aerosol treatment with isoproterenol?

a) cardiogenic pulmonary edema

b) status asthmaticus

c) IRDS

d) smoke inhalation

e) RSV pneumonia

33. Which of the following bronchodilators directly stimulates intracellular production of cAMP?

I. ipratropium bromide

II. albuterol

III. isoproterenol

IV. beclomethasone

V. metaproterenol

a) I and IV only

b) II and V only

c) II, III, and IV only

d) II, III, and V only

e) I, II, III, and V only

34. Which of the following statements are true regarding the current role of xanthines in the management of chronic asthma?

a) Xanthines are the most effective long-duration bronchodilators available.

b) Xanthines have very few side effects and the therapeutic range is easily maintained.

c) Xanthines are considered to be the most rapidly acting bronchodilators and have no cardiac side effects.

d) Xanthine use is being evaluated and in many cases discontinued in favor of mast cell stabilizers.

e) All of the above are correct.

35. Which of the following adrenergic drugs have α effects?

a) isoproterenol, metaproterenol, and albuterol

b) epinephrine, racemic peinephrine, and isoetharine

c) epinephrine and racemic epinephrine

d) pirbuterol and epinephrine

e) terbutaline, pirbuterol, and racemic epinephrine

36. Which of the following is indicated for aerosol delivery in the treatment of pneumonia caused by respiratory syncytial virus?

a) Virazole®

b) pentamidine

c) cromolyn sodium

d) ribavirin

e) both a and d

37. Which of the following drugs are aerosolized continuously into an enclosure over 8 to 12 hours by use of the SPAG nebulizer?

a) ribavirin only

b) ribavirin and pentamidine

c) colistin only

d) colistin and pentamidine

e) colistin, ribavirin, and pentamidine

38. Which of the following is *not* an advantage of aerosolizing antimicrobial drugs?

a) Scavenger systems are not needed for capturing exhaled or excess nebulized antimicrobial.

b) Bronchospasm is an extremely rare side effect.

c) Systemic side effects of the antimicrobial are eliminated.

d) Nosocomial infections may be reduced.

e) The delivery of a specific amount of drug directly to the infected site is assured.

39. Which of the following statement is the *most true* regarding the use of aerosolized antimicrobials?

a) Most FDA-approved antimicrobials are suitable and approved for aerosol delivery.

b) Aerosolizing antimicrobials is the most reliable method of assuring dosage in the patient with a pulmonary infection.

c) Many FDA-approved antimicrobials are not approved for aerosol delivery but may be appropriately aerosolized if experimental protocols are established.

d) The only drug that is FDA-approved for aerosolization is ribavirin.

e) Aerosol use of antibiotics for cystic fibrosis patients is the only FDA-approved use of aerosolized antimicrobials.

40. Cromolyn sodium and nedocromil sodium are:

a) Different brand names of the same drug, which is an antihistamine.

b) Different drugs; both exhibit mast cell stabilizing properties.

c) Different brand names of the same drug, which is an anti-inflammatory agent.

d) Antimicrobials marketed under different brand names in the United States and Canada.

e) None of the above are correct.

41. The drug of choice in the emergency treatment of croup is:

a) albuterol

b) pirbuterol

c) beclomethasone

d) cromolyn sodium

e) racemic epinephrine

42. The use of inhaled corticosteroids in the management of asthma:

a) has eliminated the need to use anticholinergic drugs.

b) emphasizes the management of the inflammation associated with asthma.

c) is only effective if used in conjunction with xanthines and systemic corticosteroids.

d) can be stopped abruptly without the need to taper dosage.

e) both b and d are correct.

43. Which of the following statements regarding surfactant-replacement drugs are true?

I. They are administered by aerosol.

II. They may be aerosolized or instilled with equal effectiveness.

III. They must be instilled directly via endotrachael tube.

IV. They are recommended for use only in the premature newborn who presents with an Apgar score less than 5 within 1 minute of delivery.

V. They are recommended for use in the premature newborn whose birthweight is less than 1500 grams or in the newborn who develops signs of IRDS.

a) III and V only

b) I, II, and V only

c) III only

d) II and IV only

e) II and V only

44. Bradycardia and oxygen desaturation are possible side effects that may occur following or during surfactant-replacement therapy with the following frequency:

a) extremely rarely.

b) rarely.

c) seldom.

d) often.

e) usually.

45. If a neonate experiences bradycardia or oxygen desaturation during administration of surfactant-replacement drugs:

a) the procedure should be interrupted and the infant stabilized; then procedure may be continued.

b) the procedure should be terminated and it should be noted that an idiosyncratic response has occurred.

c) the procedure should be completed without interruption; these are normal side effects and should not cause concern.

d) the procedure should be interrupted until the infant is stabilized; then complete the procedure using a dilute dosage and a bronchodilator.

e) none of the above.

46. Aerosolized ethyl alcohol may be considered an adjunct in the treatment of:

a) croup.

b) status asthmaticus.

c) smoke inhalation.

d) *pneumocystis carinii* pneumonia.

e) fulminant alveolar pulmonary edema.

47. Isoproterenol is occasionally used during cardiac resuscitation for which of the following purposes?

I. to increase myocardial oxygen consumption

II. to increase intracellular levels of cAMP

III. as a pharmacologic pacemaker (increase heart rate)

IV. as a potent bronchodilator

V. as a vasopressor

a) I and III only

b) II and IV only

c) III only

d) I and V only

e) I, II and IV only

48. Which of the following statements is true regarding pediatric drug dosages?

a) There are established pediatric dosages for approximately 75% of the currently FDA-approved drugs.

b) Initial pediatric drug dosage can be estimated by use of Young's Rule.

c) Initial pediatric drug dosages can be estimated by giving 50% of the recommended adult dosage.

d) It is generally not necessary to adjust drug dosages unless the patient is under 2 years of age.

e) None of the above is correct.

49. Lidocaine is administered in cardiac care for which of the following drug actions?

a) antitussive

b) local anesthetic

c) vasoconstrictor

d) anti-arrhythmic

e) beta blocker

50. Atropine is administered during cardiac resuscitation for which of the following drug actions?

a) drying of secretions

b) increased myocardial contractility

c) anti-arrhythmic

d) bronchodilator

e) calcium channel blocker

Comprehensive Exam Key

1. c
d
b
a
2. c
a
d
b
3. d
4. c
5. d
6. a
7. c
8. d
9. c
10. e
a
d
b
c
11. b
12. c
13. b
14. b
d
a
c
15. d
16. a
17. c
18. a
19. b
c
a
20. c
21. b
22. d
c
a
e
b
23. d
a
b
c
24. c
25. b
26. e
27. d
28. a
29. b
30. c
31. e
32. b
33. d
34. d
35. c
36. e
37. a
38. c
39. c
40. b
41. e
42. b
43. a
44. d
45. a
46. e
47. c
48. b
49. d
50. b